The Divine Diet: Eating To Stay Healthy

Andrew Stevens

Table of Contents

Chapter 1: The Garden of Eden

The Garden of Eden is the mythical paradise on earth that was created by God for his first two human creations, Adam and Eve. According to some, the name "Eden" is derived from the Akkadian word "plain" (ending). The garden is often referred to as the "Garden of God" because, in the biblical tradition, the biblical writers frequently mention it as a lavish location.

Our focus here, however, is on the biblical notion of a garden. The first man made in God's likeness was named Adam. God put

Adam to sleep after deciding that his loneliness was "not good" and then made Eve (the first woman) from one of Adam's ribs serve as his helper (Genesis 2:20-23). It's crucial to identify the garden's setting, the people who participated in it, and what transpired there to comprehend what the garden represents to the narrator of Genesis. All of these help us grasp what the Bible means when it refers to the "Garden of Eden."

Genesis 2:4b–3:24 in the Bible, which tells the story of Eden, puts the garden on the east side of the island. The Hebrew text contains "gan-been," which is not in the construct form, and the preposition "be" in "Weeden" is to be translated as "in." Most translations of "Garden of Eden" use the constructed element "of,"

while the Hebrew text has "gan-beeden,"
which is not in the construct form.

Therefore, translating "gan-beeden" as
"Garden of Eden" rather than "Garden in
Eden" is grammatically erroneous.
Although historians disagree on Eden's
exact location, many of them have
concluded that the garden was an alien
settlement where the gods formerly lived.

The Tigris and Euphrates rivers, which
were well-known in ancient Mesopotamia
for the creation of irrigation systems in the
surrounding region, were fed by the water
from the garden. Then, its location should
be assigned to Mesopotamia.

Place & Features

According to Genesis 2:10–14, which describes the garden, the water from Eden irrigated four significant regions: Pishon, which flows into the country of Havilah; Gihon, which flows into the land of Cush; Tigris, which runs onto Assyria's eastern side; and the fourth is the Euphrates. "Every tree that is attractive to the eye and beneficial for food" is supposed to be present in the garden. The "Tree of Life" at the garden's center and the "Tree of Knowledge of Good and Evil" are the only two trees mentioned.

The Genesis story is, however, contradictory in places. For example, Genesis 2:8–9; 3:1–3 place both trees in the middle of the garden, whereas Genesis 3:22–24 suggests that both trees may have been planted on the east side of the garden, which is where Adam was initially positioned.

Furthermore, other biblical writings that make references to the garden do not quite match the way the garden is described in the Genesis story. For instance, in Genesis 2:4b-3:24, the luxurious goods seen in the garden are not described. However, they are in Ezekiel 28. For some of these reasons, the idea of a god(s)' "garden" was a highly typical metaphor for the place where the god(s) dwelt in the ancient Near East.

The "Garden in Eden" was fictitiously created by the narrator of Genesis for an etiological (the origin or cause of things) purpose, not as a place for God to live, but rather for Adam and Eve, the first man and woman of the earth. Genesis 1–11 is referred to as the "Primeval History," which comprises mythology and traditions that were quite prevalent not only in Israel but across the ancient Near East, as is universally acknowledged in the current study.

These myths and tales are not Israelite in origin; rather, the biblical authors modified them for rhetorical or polemical effects.

To accurately understand the "Garden in Eden," readers need to consider several important issues, including What does the Genesis account of Eden serves to accomplish? What was the narrator trying to accomplish? To do this, readers mustn't approach the story's main characters—God, Adam, Eve, the snake, the two trees that are specifically mentioned—the tree of life and the tree of the knowledge of good and evil—and particularly the narrator's overarching objective.

It would be counterproductive to the narrative's storyline to concentrate just on the "garden" while ignoring these folks.

EARLY INFLUENCE

Ancient literature often used symbols and metaphors; these devices include rhetorical devices intended to convince readers to accept the information being delivered. In other words, the literature of antiquity had a purpose. Works give anything or something its complete expression.

According to the oldest known literature that is credited to the Sumerians, myths about the place of a god's (or gods') home in the ancient Near East often take place in gardens. In Genesis, God puts Adam and Eve in the garden of Eden rather than staying there. This is sufficient to show readers how the narrator of Genesis adapted the garden idea, which interpreters often overlook.

The lower Tigris-Euphrates Valley was home to the Sumerians, a highly talented non-Semitic group of uncertain ancestry that arrived there during the fourth millennium BC.

The lovely island of Dilmun seems to resemble the Christian idea of heaven, where life never ends, based on the little description provided. There is no mention of old age on the island or in the country, which is said to be "pure," "clean," and "bright." According to Sumerian literature, the sun deity Utu raised this island or piece of land from the ground and transformed it into a true garden of the gods. It seems that the garden (Dilmun) in Sumerian myth was a location created by a deity or gods for gods.

VERSION IN GENESIS

The narrator of the book of Genesis undoubtedly used the Sumerian literary idea of a garden as an otherworldly location for theological and etiological objectives. One must study the setting and individuals involved in the story—God, the Garden of Eden, Adam, Eve, the serpent, and the two trees—to comprehend

Genesis' depiction of the garden (tree of life and tree of knowledge).

The Dilmun Island was modified by the Genesis storyteller to fit his/her/their audience's objective. However, in the Genesis account, God simply declared that there would be death and issues between God and humankind as a consequence of Adam and Eve's intentional act of eating the fruit from the forbidding "tree of knowledge." The Garden of Eden was a paradise of unending delight free from death, much like the country of Dilmun. Adam and Eve disobeyed God by trying to become gods, and as a response, God secured the "tree of life" by embedding cherubim with flaming swords to block access to it. Another significant improvement made by the Genesis narrator of the Dilmun Island

God doesn't live in the garden; he puts Adam and Eve there. Theologically speaking, it should be noted that, in contrast to other gods, the God of Genesis intended to build a connection with humans.

In the book of Genesis, the Eden story serves one of two purposes, to put it simply. First, the creation tale in Genesis 1:1–2:4a, which concludes with the words: "And God saw everything that he had created, and behold, it was very good," comes before the Eden narrative. The Eden story contrasts the completed creation as "very good" with disruption (Adam and Eve's disobedience in Genesis 2:4b-3:24), painting a picture of the completed creation as "very good" with disruption. Readers can easily forget that

God had planted the "Tree of Life" and the "Tree of Knowledge," two unique trees, in the middle of the garden. The "Tree of Knowledge" has received more focus than the "Tree of Life."

The "Tree of Life" is mentioned and has a significant purpose in the story. The sole fruit from the "tree of knowledge" that God forbade Adam and Eve from eating. Why did God not stop Adam and Eve from eating from the "tree of life" is a crucial issue. They were not to eat from any trees, except for the "Tree of Knowledge," according to God's instructions (Gen. 2:16-17).

The "tree of life" was also available for Adam and Eve to eat, but they instead choose to reject God's instruction, according to the narrator of the Eden tale.

According to the narrator, evil has infiltrated the universe that was intended to be "very good" as a result of Adam and Eve's arrogance to become gods.

The audience that the storyteller is trying to reach must decide between life (obedience) and death (disobedience). Adam and Eve's transgression caused a breakdown in God's relationship with mankind. The world that Adam and Eve, not God, created as "very good" now contains death or evil (as a concept). Humans produce evil.

Second, the Eden story also serves as an etiological mythology that seeks to explain the origin of humans. Genesis 1:1–2:4a's account of creation has previously answered problems about the cosmogony, which was God's creation. According to the story of Eden, Adam and Eve were the first humans and the first parents who created mankind.

The Eden narrative is intended to make conjectures about the beginnings of mankind and its original home, much like cosmogonic literature from the ancient Near East. It seems that the "Primeval History" part of Genesis contains myths concerning the origins of human knowledge, which would naturally conflict with scientific findings made in the twenty-first century CE.

CONCLUSION

The first place that God gave to humans was the Garden of Eden. In contrast to Sumerian traditions, God did not build the Garden of Eden for himself, but rather for

Adam and Eve. God is not portrayed by the narrator as being self-centered but rather as loving.

According to Genesis, God's divine position was exalted to the point where He no longer required a corporeal home since doing so would only compromise His omnipresence. According to the interpretation above, the Garden in Eden is a garden "in" Eden rather than a garden "of" Eden. Based on the Hebrew translation of "gan-beeden" that was previously offered, this assumes that this specific garden was maybe not the only one in Eden.

Chapter 2: God's Original Diet In The Garden

Did you realize that Genesis 1:29 contains information on God's initial diet? "Behold, I have given you every plant that has fruit that is on the face of the whole world, and every tree that bears fruit that bears seed; you shall eat of it."

God instructed Adam and Eve to follow a diet of the most basic sort, which He supplied for them, and placed them in a garden. Their meal consisted of the tree's fruits and flowering plants that produced seeds. God provided the food that He intended for the race to consume to our ancestors. To have the life of any creature snatched was against His design. In Eden, there would be no death. The sustenance needed by man was found in the garden's fruit-bearing trees.

The Bible also states that when Adam's transgression caused him to be expelled from the Garden of Eden, God gave him instructions to modify the diet described in Genesis 1:29 to include "herb of the field" (see Genesis 3:18). Because Adam had been denied access to the Tree of Life, which offered immortality, vegetables, and other garden herbs were added to the original living food scheme. Because Adam may have now required the additional vitamins and minerals offered by the plants that grew on the land, the veggies were included in God's health regimen.

In particular, chlorophyll, or concentrated solar power, which is similar to hemoglobin in red blood cells, was contributed by these new meals. Green vegetables are excellent blood builders and may turn green blood in plants into red blood in people. Yes, God created phytochemical-rich vegetables to support the body's immune system and keep Adam and Eve healthy.

Because they are grown in the same soil that man was created from, vegetables are abundant in nutrients including calcium, magnesium, potassium, and trace minerals. Vegetables are a good source of protein and vitamins, including vitamins A, B, and C.

We are animate organisms that are sustained by earth-grown live plants.

Plants are nutrient- and calorie-rich high-octane fuel that God created to power and mend the human body. By consuming the plants He has made and allowed to flourish on the ground, we remineralize ourselves.

Another argument is that because you and I were created after sin, we need fruits, nuts, grains, and vegetables to produce healthy blood. "It is erroneous to believe that the consumption of animal products is necessary for the development of physical strength. Without it, the system's demands may be better met, and more robust health can be experienced.

All the nutritional components required to produce healthy blood are included in the grains, along with fruits, nuts, and vegetables. A diet high in meat does not adequately or entirely provide these nutrients. Animal food would have been a part of the diet that was prescribed to man in the beginning if eating flesh had been necessary for health and vigor.

The next catastrophe, the Great Flood, called for a temporary but essential change to the all-plant diet described in Genesis 1:29 and 3:18. Every moving creature that lives shall be meat for you; exactly as the green herb have I given you all things after the Great Flood in Noah's day when God changed the original diet plan and added flesh to man's diet.

God originally allowed His people permission to eat the flesh of dead animals, but never the blood or the fat: "But flesh with the life thereof, which is the blood thereof, shalt ye not eat." This was after all living creatures were wiped off the face of the world (see Genesis 7:21–23). 9:4 in Genesis We must recognize that God provided particular dietary guidelines on which animals may be consumed and which could not as part of the temporary diet of eating flesh (see Leviticus 11 for the clean and unclean list).

But given that plant foods are so readily accessible nowadays and can be found at any supermarket or, even better, picked fresh from one's garden, must we still adhere to the temporary diet? "If there was ever a period when the diet should be the simplest possible kind, this is it. Our youngsters shouldn't be served meat. Its effect is to stir up and bolster the baser emotions, and it tends to weaken moral faculties. The meal on the tables of everyone who claims to be preparing for translation to heaven should be grains and fruits, as natural as possible (there is nothing more natural than raw).

According to a different remark, "God is restoring His people to His original plan, which is to not eat the flesh of dead animals, as I have repeatedly shown. He wanted us to show others how to do things better. By "His original plan," what does God mean? Our research makes it clear that He is referring to a vegan diet that excludes all animal products, as described in Genesis 1:29 and 3:18.

In addition, the SOP has one additional phrase that challenges us to return to His original plan: "Let our people eliminate all unwholesome recipes. Let them gain knowledge about healthy living and pass it on to others. Let them share this information as they would a lesson from the Bible. Let them instruct the populace on how to strengthen themselves and maintain their health by avoiding the excessive cooking that has caused so many chronically sick individuals to populate the planet. Make it clear via example and precept that the food that God provided for Adam in his sinless condition is the finest for man to eat as he strives to become sinless once again.

Since there was neither a fire for cooking in Eden nor any death, the phrase "in his sinless condition" implies that Adam's diet consisted exclusively of living food before he ate the forbidden fruit and sinned. The first animal wasn't killed until after he was chased out of the garden (see Genesis 3:21). Since we were born after sin and must eat veggies, I don't believe it implies to be a fruitarian, but it could be suggesting to consume your food in the same manner that Adam did—alive! In the "sinless condition," live and uncooked foods were constantly consumed. When you suggest or encourage someone to pursue a 100% raw food diet, some individuals take offense. If you're one of them, consider this: "Will the diet God provided our original parents in Eden remain the same on the new earth? Will cooking even cause death in Eden Restored?

According to the Bible and the Spirit of Prophecy, the heavenly Canaan will be bountiful with living food and, as in Eden, without the need for vegetables once again since we will all be living sinlessly. The Tree of Life, which "bore twelve sorts of

fruits, and produced her fruit every month"
(see Revelation 22:2), bestowed its bounty
once again to the seer John in a vision.

There are a ton of wonderful raw food
recipes! Because cooking food over 115
degrees kills enzymes, raw and live foods
are preferable to prepared ones. The living
enzymes in grains and seeds may be
preserved by learning how to sprout them.
Additionally, heating food may alter its
molecular structure and, in certain
situations, make it hazardous; microwave
cooking is the worst. Living foods often
offer more nutritional content than cooked
meals and more antioxidants to stave
against illness.

Please understand that I am not advocating
that everyone consumes just raw foods or
abstain from all forms of cooking; that is

entirely up to you. But I have to say that I now value a raw diet or at least one that has a lot of live food, as being the healthiest for people today. "Health reform is an informed selection of the most nutritious piece of food served in the most beneficial, simplest manner," said Dr. Mercola.

"The Lord wishes to restore His people to a life of basic fruits, vegetables, and grains; God gave the fruit to our first parents in its original condition."

God is advancing the interests of His people. He does not want them to need anything. He is reintroducing them to the diet that was first prescribed to man. Their diet should only include items created from the ingredients He has given them. Use basic, unprocessed ingredients that are as near to nature as possible while cooking, free of chemicals and pesticides, and always fresh.

The electrical charge in the living foods charges us when we consume them. They have greater energy, a calmer stomach, a lighter demeanor, and sleep better at night if they avoid consuming cooked protein meals, which need big stomach acid production and might cause GERD or acid reflux. Many individuals who consume raw foods follow a low-protein diet and don't have any gastrointestinal issues. For those who wish to reduce weight, the diet is excellent.

As promised in Deuteronomy 7:14 and 15, we think God wants His distinctive people to be the healthiest people on earth. "Thou will be blessed above all people:... And the

LORD will remove all illness from thee, and he will not inflict any bad diseases upon thee."

Have you ever considered the seven-year diet of only grass that King Nebuchadnezzar followed, according to Daniel 4:32?

In Daniel Chapter 1, Daniel and his three companions reject the king's diet of meat and wine and choose to consume only complete plant foods, veganism, and clean water instead. This suggests that King Nebuchadnezzar must have had a diet heavy in protein and fat for most of his life as it was the king's meat and drink. It is reasonable to infer that the King was very poisonous and may have had occasional constipation as a result of the feasts that included no fiber. He undoubtedly raised his chances of developing colon cancer.

The monarch deserved to be humiliated in addition to being unwell. He was, after all, the King of Babylon and was revered as a deity. He had a pride issue, according to the Bible. According to Daniel chapter 3, he ruled that everyone present at the dedication of the golden image had to kneel before the image of gold, which stood in for Nebuchadnezzar and Babylon.

Anyone who didn't pay respect to the monarch would be thrown into a blazing fire. The three Hebrews were tossed into the seven-times-hotter-than-normal fire for their refusal to submit to the human potentate. Even though he had only thrown three men into the fire, the king saw a fourth one there whom he compares to the Son of God, Jesus. Despite the incredible circumstances, not a hair on their heads was damaged. The converted king then honors the God of Shadrach, Meshach, and Abednego and orders the whole country to acknowledge the real God.

We read that Nebuchadnezzar reverses course and is once again elevated to the status of a deity in Daniel Chapter 4. The haughty king would now be driven away from people to eat grass among the animals of the field by the real God of the Hebrews. "Thy home shall be with the animals of the field; they shall make thee eat grass as oxen, and seven times [years] shall pass over thee," said the prophet Daniel, "till thou knowest that the Highest ruleth in the kingdom of mankind, and giveth it to whomsoever He will." Dan. 4:32.

When you think that King Nebuchadnezzar survived for seven years on nothing but grass, the tale is incredibly intriguing. It's possible to wonder: "Is that even feasible?

Let's examine the grass known as wheatgrass. Barley grass and wheatgrass are two of the best sources of vitamins A, B, and C, and they are quite similar to one another. They are also quite mineral-rich. They serve as a body cleanser, builder, and toxin neutralizer. Even radiation protection is provided by these plants.

The nutritious content of 1 pound of wheatgrass is equivalent to approximately 25 pounds of the finest vegetables, claims

Ann Wigmore. She also claimed that wheatgrass treatment assisted in treating a variety of illnesses, including mental problems, and helped to remove malignant growths. Very successful in curing anemia.

Wheatgrass has a lot of concentrated solar energy called chlorophyll. For both internal and external ailments, it is one of the best healers. It builds and purifies the blood. It boosts red cell production, cleanses the liver, treats blood sugar issues, and hastens wound healing. In the bloodstream, it functions like a detergent.

Fresh juices are blood builders and healers. They are abundant in enzymes, which are the sparks of life, vitamins, minerals, and trace elements.

The circulation and cells can absorb almost all of the essential nutrients without placing undue stress on the digestive system. Juices revitalize the body, hastening its recovery from illness. Since over-acidity affects so many Americans today, these alkaline foods are excellent for regulating pH. The prevalence of acid reflux is increasing and it is a generational illness. With all the acid-forming foods like meat, dairy, alcohol, coffee, and sugar, the GI tract is suffering.

Juices provide abundant levels of minerals like calcium, potassium, and silicon that are simple to absorb since they are in liquid form and, as a result, help to restore the balance of minerals in the cells. They may restore pH equilibrium since they are meals that produce alkali.

Natural antibiotics, hormones, and phytochemicals are found in raw juices. For diabetics, Jerusalem artichokes and string beans have compounds that resemble insulin. The pancreatic cells require hormone-like compounds in onions and cucumbers to create insulin. Natural antibiotics may be found in radishes, garlic, and onions.

Plants' vibrant reds, yellows, greens, and blue hues all contain phytochemicals that ward against and combat cancer.

Apple juice contains pectin, which binds to heavy metals and cleanses the intestines of impurities.

High in nutrients, beet juice purifies and strengthens the blood as well as detoxifies the liver.

The cleansing sulfur and vitamin C in cabbage juice are abundant. Vitamin U is present for stomach ulcers.

Celery juice helps calm the nervous system and neutralizes acid with its organic sodium thanks to its mineral composition.

Juiced dandelion greens promote bile flow and aid in liver and gallbladder cleansing.

Beta carotene, chlorophyll, calcium, and iron are all abundant in kale juice.

Beta carotene, chlorophyll, and vitamin and mineral-rich parsley juice have diuretic and great blood-cleansing qualities.

All green juices are packed with antioxidants and are excellent for boosting blood production and overall health. They are excellent for low blood levels and anemia.

Given the healing potential of green, it seems to sense that God would have chosen that food to save the monarch's life while also humbling the king. But given the detoxifying properties of green grass, it is not unexpected that King Nebuchadnezzar's reason and comprehension returned after seven years of just eating green grass, and he exalted, worshipped, and worshiped the "King of heaven." Dan. 4:27.

Here are some recipes for green smoothies that you may try. Smoothies made of greens are incredibly nourishing and

simple to digest. a tasty method to get
veggies into your kids.

Combine the following ingredients.

Lemon, Kale, and Apple: 4 apples
1/2 lemon (juice only) 5 kale leaves
(remove white stems for better taste)
2-cups of water

Six peaches and six spinach leaves
Twice as much spinach
2 glasses of water

Pear, Chard, and Mint: 4 ripe pears, 5
chard leaves
12 bundles of mint
2-cups of water

Chapter 3: God's Interest In Your Health

We often take our health for granted until we start to deteriorate. When our health declines, we immediately start to doubt our routines and nutrition. God created the human body to be the most robust instrument on earth and a highly tuned instrument. It can withstand adhesions and fractures, ongoing discomfort, and lengthy periods of boredom.

It is a delicate instrument, however, since it was not intended to manage excess, whether it comes in the form of fuel, food, or additives. It chokes on toxins when swallowed in endless amounts and is misidentified as fuel, unlike machines. Despite having movement, feeling, and cognitive components, these elements may be abused. God has given us an "owner's handbook" that explains how the human body functions. The Bible is that guidebook, a book with guidelines for good upkeep. God's Word, while not a medical manual, contains many fundamental guidelines for optimum bodily, mental, and spiritual health.

Moses was responsible for most of the biblical guidance on health. However, many scientists and physicians today are astounded by the precision and potency of its many provisions.

According to the Wycliffe Bible Encyclopedia, God gave Moses regulations that include outstanding guidelines for public health issues that still worry us today, such as water and food pollution, sewage disposal, contagious illnesses, and health education. The Mosaic health laws addressed each of these concerns.

The fundamental secret to good bodily and mental health is revealed in the Bible. The answer is in the following simple statement: "My son, do not forget my instruction, but retain my precepts in your heart because they will lengthen your life many years and bring you riches. Your body will benefit from this and your bones will get nutrients (Proverbs 3:1-2, 8).

We shouldn't be surprised that following God's instructions and other rules will improve our health. We function in conformity with His directives when we obey them. He understands what's best for us since He's our Creator: "Now that everything has been spoken, this is the judgment: Fear God and obey his commands because this is the whole obligation of man" (Ecclesiastes 12:13).

Specific biblical verses about health include: "I will not bring on you any of the diseases I brought on the Egyptians, for I am the LORD, who heals you," and "If you pay careful attention to the voice of the LORD your God and do what is right in his eyes, if you pay attention to his commands and keep all his decrees" (Exodus 15:26).

The illnesses that have plagued humanity throughout history affected the ancient Egyptians. Evidence of smallpox, arteriosclerosis, cancer, arthritis, gallstones, bladder stones, TB, and other ailments have been found during autopsies on Egyptian mummies. They were afflicted with several illnesses as a result of their ignorance of the health guidelines God imparted to Moses.

The application of cause-and-effect principles, which are based on real science, is required in the biblical instructions for maintaining health and recovering from illness. These instructions were given thousands of years before scientists had the technology to discover germs, bacteria, viruses, genes, and the like. Many elements of good health have been discovered by modern medical research, but they were first discovered by God, who designed and constructed the miraculous human body.

According to what the Bible states, those who follow God will often be in good health. The implication is not necessarily that individuals who reject God will always be unwell. Furthermore, it does not imply that God's people would be completely immune from illness. "I hope that you may have excellent health and that things may go well with you, even as your soul is getting along well," the Bible states (3 John 1:2). God obviously cares more about our spiritual health than our physical health, but He also wants us to be well physically. However, because of Adam's fall, sickness exists, and even the most upright people may become sick. Job was righteous after all, but God permitted him to experience sickness and adversity.

Men did not have an in-depth understanding of human physiology and medicine until the contemporary age. But the Creator God often referred to as the

Great Physician, is well aware of our circumstances and has given us the tools we need to maintain good health. We have the option to obey the Lord and enjoy the rewards that follow.

Chapter 4: The Health Benefits of The Garden of Eden Diet

What did God eat in the Garden of Eden at first? Fruits, grains, nuts, and legumes are mentioned in Genesis as food groups. God made the "herb of the field" veggies after sin.

According to the Bible, God provided the Eden diet:

And God said, "Behold, I have given you every plant producing seed found on the surface of the world, as well as every tree bearing fruit from a plant bearing seed,

which you shall use for sustenance"
(Genesis 1:29).

The Eden diet, often known as the first
human diet, was a vegetarian diet
consisting of fruits, grains, and nuts.

After people sinned and were barred from
the tree of life, God introduced vegetables
to the human diet. Every living creature
that moves will be food for you;
everything has been provided to you like a
green plant (Genesis 9:3). Man was also
permitted to consume the clean animal
meat specified in (Deut. 14 and Leviticus
11).

After then, it took more than 12 generations for the life expectancy of a man to drop from 900 to around 120 years. This was caused in part by the introduction of animal products soon after the flood, the rise of cooking, and the decline in the consumption of green vegetation.

And why do people nowadays not live to be 120 years old? There was presumably a progressive growth in the cooking of vegetables and fruits along with the cooking of meat. Fresh fruits and vegetables lose some of their nutritional value when they are cooked. The majority of the food in our diet nowadays is either cooked or processed, and it contains a lot of animal products, some of which may be

unhealthy because of their high-fat
content.

We also consume a little bit of uncooked
green plants at the same time. The ideal
healthy diet that God designed is not this
one. Weak immune systems, illness, early
aging, and death are the final results.

Naturally, a vegetarian diet is the best diet.
It is the first diet. However, individuals
must arrange a well-balanced mix of
various meals while following the
vegetarian diet to receive all the necessary
elements for optimal health.

A full diet includes enough fiber, vitamins
C and E, folic acid, magnesium,
unsaturated fat, and a wide variety of

phytochemicals. And this explains why vegetarians have lower blood pressure, cholesterol, and a decreased chance of developing heart disease. Additionally, vegetarian cuisine is simple to prepare, quick to digest, healthful, and most significantly, economical. In addition to being essential for a healthy lifestyle, vegetables also benefit the environment.

Benefits of Eating Vegetarian
Here are 10 incredible advantages of becoming a vegetarian.

1. Lengthens the lifetime

Although many other variables might contribute to a longer lifespan, one thing you can follow is to adopt a vegetarian diet. The more fruits and vegetables you consume, the fewer toxins and chemicals accumulate in your body, allowing you to live a longer, healthier life.

2. Lower levels of cholesterol

Whether you want to believe it or not, consuming animal fat has no health benefits. Vegetarian diets are cholesterol-free since only animal products contain cholesterol. Although cholesterol is a necessary component of every human cell, vegetarians do not need to be concerned about receiving adequate cholesterol since vegan diets provide the body with all the cholesterol it requires.

After looking at the long-term consequences of eating a vegetarian diet,

Korean researchers concluded that vegetarians have lower levels of body fat and cholesterol than omnivores.

3. Reduced risk of obesity and stroke

Vegetarians often make considerably more thoughtful meal selections and seldom overeat or make emotional eating decisions, two habits that significantly increase the risk of obesity.

Adopting a vegan diet is recommended as a smart method to reduce your risk of developing a stroke or becoming fat, according to the pediatrics department of the University Hospital Ghent in Belgium.

4. Decreases diabetes risk

Non-vegetarians often have very high blood sugar levels just after eating, sometimes even very high levels. If non-vegetarians go on a vegetarian diet, this may be prevented and a steady flow of blood sugar can be maintained. A healthful vegetarian diet that is also simple to digest has fewer fatty acids.

5. Provides wholesome skin

You must consume the proper ratio of vitamins and minerals together with lots of water if you want to have good skin. The fruits and vegetables we consume are particularly high in vitamins, minerals, and antioxidants.

Additionally, because they are water-based, eating them uncooked might increase your intake of beneficial elements. Numerous vegetarian meals are also abundant in antioxidants, which support healthy skin and a long life free of illness.

6. A high amount of fiber

High fiber content is also present in fruits and vegetables, which is essential for healthy digestion. It aids in enhancing body metabolism and speeds up the removal of toxins and other substances from

your body. The majority of vegetarian diets are water-based, which aids in maintaining the body's necessary fluid balance.

7. Can help with depression.

Vegetarians may be happier than their non-vegetarian colleagues, according to studies. Additionally, it was shown that vegans performed better on depression tests and mood profiles than meat- or fish-eaters. Additionally, most vegetarian dishes include a freshness component, particularly when it comes to organic fruit. It will thus undoubtedly purify our brains and maintain their positivity.

8. Enhances metabolism

Vegetarian cuisine is simple to digest and helps people maintain a healthy metabolism. Additionally, vegetarians have far greater RMRs than nonvegetarians do. You should be aware that an individual's metabolism and RMR are directly related; the greater the RMR, the faster the body burns fat; and vice versa.

9. Lowers the possibility of developing cataracts

The chance of acquiring cataracts is strongly correlated with our diet, with nonvegetarians and meat eaters having a greater risk and vegans having the lowest risk, according to a study from the University of Oxford's Nuffield Department of Clinical Medicine.

10. It is affordable

Last but not least, eating a vegetarian diet allows you to save a significant sum of

money. Without a doubt, non-vegetarian
food is more costly than vegetarian food.
The decision is now entirely up to you.

You must incorporate these vegetarian
foods into your diet:

- Beans

- Lentils

- Nuts

- Veggies with leaves, etc.

To sum up, there are a lot more advantages
to eating vegetarian cuisine than what we
have covered in this post. Additionally, we
don't want to denigrate or belittle

non-vegetarians. Both vegetarian and
non-vegetarian cuisine offer advantages.

Stay Healthy by Eating Well!

Chapter 5: It Is A Choice To Stay Healthy

Your body's continuous health and vitality, assuming you were born with a functional one that hasn't been damaged by an accident or injury, are a matter of decision. Some interrelated components and related, crucial actions are necessary for maintaining health. For the advantages of any one of them to be fully realized, they must all be in place. These are a few of them:

Keep your intestines in good shape.

- eating the proper, whole foods to provide your body with what it requires.

- As your body's main source of fuel, burn fat.

- avoiding toxicity in food and the surroundings where one life.

- Avoid using your phone too much and EMFs.

- Physical activity and workout.

- consuming enough clean water. Along with basic hygiene

- obtaining enough, high-quality sleep.

- Spending time outdoors will keep you connected to the planet, in a healthy ecosystem, and the sunlight.

- Regular fasting

Using a stress-reduction technique for
health

To the degree that these things can be
controlled, choosing your health is a
decision. In addition to the difficulty and
expense of obtaining clean water, new
parents may first have difficulty sleeping
through the night. You will struggle to
keep your vitamin D levels at their ideal
levels in the winter at latitudes farther
north than southern France.

Consider the option of long- or
medium-term planning, however, to put all
of these variables within your control.
Because lifestyle decisions have an impact
on health, plan your whole lifestyle around
maintaining good health. Any lifestyle
decision that compromises your health,

including the foods you consume, is not a good idea in the long run. For instance, choosing health is not compatible with shift employment that prevents proper sleep.

Training for health

Your health is mostly a result of "knowing what to do" to maintain it. Humans do not have a natural understanding of which foods to consume or which toxins to avoid. People did not aware until very recently in human history that access to clean water and minimum hygiene standards are prerequisites for health; now, we take these things for granted. Like that, our understanding of germ theory, viruses, bacteria, and the part they play in infection and the transmission of illness is likewise rather young in comparison to our evolutionary history.

Either you can think for yourself and make your own decisions, or you may mimic people around you to understand what is necessary for health (or anything else, for that matter). Thought has always been the path to knowledge, the initial approach hasn't always been as dangerous as it is today. Due to two key factors, the context has shifted.

First off, since the industrial revolution, we have had more options than most people can fathom. In the past, there was no such option, and health results were mostly determined by external factors. For instance, most people ate what they could to avoid poverty, and there was no such thing as modern environmental degradation.

The second justification is crucial. Because so many individuals are doing it incorrectly, copying what others do is no longer an effective tactic! Knowledge is readily accessible since we live in the information era, yet it is all muddled together. Official recommendations that are incorrect and newly discovered knowledge that is 100% accurate point in different ways.

For instance, dietary saturated fat cannot be both good for you and bad for you. A chemical can't be both necessary for human existence and terrible for you and the root of heart disease. Mercury amalgam fillings cannot be both a risky neurotoxin and safe for your mouth. Only one of these scenarios can be true in all of them. The alternative is untrue. It is difficult to separate reality from fiction and truth from falsehood, which is why following the crowd is no longer acceptable.

Thinking independently

It takes thinking and a process of self-education to gain information. The good news is that, even though it is no longer wise to imitate others, we don't have to invent the wheel and do independent health research. But we do need to take the time to educate ourselves and make wise decisions from the vast amount of knowledge that is nowadays publicly accessible thanks to the Internet.

We must decide for ourselves. Our ability to think independently and trust our judgment is essential to maintaining our health in the modern world.

The pursuit of health will continue to seem like a lottery for individuals who lack the ability or desire to think for themselves. They won't know who to mimic or who to pay attention to to get accurate information.

consuming the proper foods

What we choose to consume is the main aspect that affects our health. According to the data, what we typically eat may put us 80% of the way on the road to health. The majority of us have total freedom of choice in this regard, therefore this is fantastic news. Children have to follow their parents' or caretakers' decisions, and those who work in institutions like hospitals often have little say in these matters. However, the majority of adults who live alone have complete discretion over what they choose to eat. It is a basic right that we all own and the most effective influencer on our health. On the other hand, contemporary research indicates that consuming improper foods is the main contributor to the majority of illnesses.

Even though we have mastered basic sanitation and access to clean water, far too many people still suffer as a result of eating incorrect foods or being exposed to toxins found in those foods or the environment.

The vast majority of the foods in today's shops will jeopardize our health yet there are infinite temptations for your taste senses. This makes ensuring a healthy choice more difficult. The problem is made more difficult by bad government guidance. This has caused the prevalence of contemporary chronic illnesses to significantly rise.

Diet is crucial for two reasons.

Your body's cells must get the nutrients they need to operate. This implies that to meet our whole range of nutritional needs, we must consume the correct foods. Over time, a diet low in any one vitamin will make you sick.

Second, there must be no toxicity that compromises any cell. Our health will suffer if we consume harmful foods and substances that shouldn't be in our bodies. Because of this, it's important to choose our food carefully. Think about toxicity and quality. By definition, food with organic certification is non-GMO and less harmful than food without one. It is a red herring to ask whether or not you can taste the difference or if there is any nutritional difference.

Some substances should be avoided since they are harmful to nature. Chemical food additives such as stabilizers, emulsifiers, binding agents, and flavor enhancers are a few examples of these. Wheat damages the stomach lining and may trigger auto-immune illnesses, in which the body starts to see a portion of itself as an invading alien body, thus there is also a good case for avoiding it.

We are unable to link nutritional inadequacy and/or toxicity and how it ultimately affects our health, so we continue to engage in poor eating habits without realizing the consequences.

Preventing toxicity in the environment and food

In the current situation, it's critical to be on the lookout for toxicity in both food and the environment. We are all capable of doing this. By not doing so, we run the risk of letting ignorance endanger our health. If one is concerned about their health, one should participate in the thought process outlined in the bullet points below.

Eating organically is, by definition, less harmful.

- Eating raw food prevents the food's nutritious value from being destroyed.

- eating grass-fed organic meats, staying away from meat from CAFOs, and drinking pasteurized milk

- A deadly soup is poured into the blood during vaccinations, and mercury from amalgam fillings drips into the intestines.

- noxious household goods

- hazardous personal care products

- electromagnetic (EMF) contamination in the air and

Poisoning ourselves while pretending to be looking for health is not acceptable.

Physical activity and workout

Exercise and physical activity are previously known to be beneficial for health. Sitting is the new smoking, and there are numerous reasons why such a sedentary lifestyle is bad. The key message is that every one of us has control over our actions and how much we decide to move and exercise. Everyone has the option to exercise.

The following is a summary of the key factors to think about while incorporating healthy activity into our life. In later postings,

- Stretching exercises, including yoga, maintain flexibility.

- aerobic activity

- exercise for muscle

- Interval training with a high (or varying) intensity

Consuming enough clean water

Drinking enough water is another aspect of health that is crucial but is often ignored. Although it takes some time to develop a new habit of being aware of this demand, it is unquestionably well within our power. Here in England, tap water should be filtered because it is so highly polluted. If you decide to buy bottled water, glass is a better option than plastic.

Obtaining enough, quality sleep

Your body requires a certain amount of sleep to operate effectively. This is for a variety of reasons, which we shall examine in a later article. The idea here is that practically all of us are capable of choosing when to go to bed so that we may have a restful night's sleep. Working the night shift is not advised since it is not long-term health-compatible.

If you work evenings and want to stay healthy, you should make plans to switch to another career that will both support your financial demands and protect your health. Even if one must work shifts for a while due to circumstances, a strategic adjustment may be planned over time.

Nutrition D

The only solution, in this case, is self-education. It is fully within our ability to learn what our bodies need if we all want to be healthy. For a variety of reasons, vitamin D is crucial to good health. You may use a specially made sun lamp or take a supplement if you reside in a latitude where you get inadequate sunlight throughout the winter. If you do take a vitamin D supplement, it's crucial to also take a vitamin K2 supplement.

Boosting your immune system is beneficial for your health.

This category contains many considerations, all of which are deserving of a thorough examination. The basis of good health is gut health. 80% of the immune system is located in the gut, and impacts mental wellness as well. Anyone who has control over their diet may affect their gut health and put the other crucial components of keeping a healthy gut into practice. One may choose to have a healthy digestive system.

It is important to understand that dental health is an integral part of our entire health. The two are often unrelated to one another. However, certain careless dental procedures might gravely harm health by poisoning the immune system.

Mercury amalgam fillings are inappropriate for use in human mouths.

The same holds for root canal procedures and any implant type that involves the introduction of metal into the mouth. This is a decision that calls for some in-depth self-education.

By reducing oxidative stress, being electrically connected to the soil also benefits the immune system. It's advised to sleep with a grounding sheet and go barefoot, and we may choose to do any of these things.

Another crucial aspect of the larger picture of health is the implementation of a stress management or reduction approach. If it is not too much, stress might be beneficial. It is within our power to make lifestyle decisions that will guarantee we have some kind of stress-relieving activities. It doesn't matter what you do—meditation, strolling, reading, whatever suits you—as long as you like it. Again, we can control this.

Periodic fasting

Since the beginning of human development, people have been fasting. Before agriculture, people living in temperate areas would have had to fast throughout the winter months out of need. It provides so many advantages because of this. Some of the outcomes include a longer lifespan, improved immunological response, and mental clarity.

Being in nutritional ketosis is a technique to replicate the fasting state and get all the advantages of fasting without the hassles and difficulties. There are many different ways to fast, including alternate day fasting, in which you eat one day and fast the next, water fasts, in which you consume only water for anywhere between one day and five days, five-day fasts, and what Dr. Joseph Mercola calls "Peak Fasting," an intermittent fasting method. I would strongly advise anybody interested in staying healthy to consider fasting as an important component of their overall health plan. The key takeaway is that we have full control over this exercise and lifestyle decision.

What matters most in life?

It's difficult to change one's lifestyle, and for certain individuals, I believe it's particularly difficult to alter one's eating habits. But since what we eat has such a significant impact on how we feel, avoiding chronic illness and promoting lifespan and health must be the major goal. It all boils down to analyzing your options and deciding what matters most. Our future dietary choices may be influenced if we intentionally determine that our health is the most essential component of our existence.

When we are striving to succeed in altering our behaviors, we are the only ones in the ring. That dragon must be slain on our own, as is often the case. Knowing what to consume and what to avoid, as well as retaining the self-discipline to carry out the ensuing plan of action, are our responsibilities. It is perhaps the most realistic endeavor for personal growth one can take on, and it has the biggest benefit: health.

The effect of a lifestyle decision is health

This implies that it relies on how we decide to live. Do we live in a manner that promotes each of the aforementioned elements necessary for good health? We cannot expect to be long-term health if we don't. Our health may be improved or harmed depending on a variety of things, including where we live, what we eat, what we do for a livelihood, how much sleep we get, the personal care products we use, and even how we wash.

These days, proactive lifestyle planning that involves deliberate consideration is beneficial to us. Simply settling into a way of life won't likely be beneficial to you. The unwatchful, unwary, or ignorant will not have the evolutionary advantage.

In general, today's population of people does not live morally. They don't strive for "proper living." The majority of patients with a typical chronic ailment will unknowingly follow the herd and end up in the hospital in the future. We will have taken a very significant first step toward healthy living if we alter our perspective and take initiative in this direction.

Decide to live a healthy lifestyle, then plan your lifestyle around that choice.

Chapter 6: God's Principles of Health

How do you maintain your health? Does your Christian life have anything to do with your health? Scripture lays forth important guidelines that might make your life longer and happier!

Is health a goal in and of itself, or is it a means to an end? How can we achieve and keep health in the contemporary world?

For many years, maintaining good health was seen as a means to an end—to help one live, make a living, raise a family, or achieve a lofty objective. Today, finding the right diet or kind of exercise to build the ideal physique has replaced seeking health as a goal in itself. Today, many people worship their bodies and their health as contemporary deities!

Millions of people look for the newest health secrets in an everlasting quest for physical perfection. Adjustments, injections, medications, and procedures cost a lot of money, even for personal trainers! Some people follow gurus.

Others search for the unique nutrient or the miraculous treatment! Americans spend more than a trillion dollars on health care each year, along with billions on supplements and complementary therapies, yet they are not the healthiest population in the world.

In the United States, the overweight rate is above 60%. Over 30% of people are fat. Heart disease, cancer, stroke, diabetes, and other illnesses affect millions of people. For mental illnesses, millions of people use medications. In other industrialized countries, the tale is similar. For many, the current, all-consuming pursuit of health is a costly, never-ending hunt for the proverbial "holy grail" that often falls short of bringing about the health and tranquility of mind that the majority of people want.

But we must inquire, "Why?" Is there a component lacking in our current understanding of health? Western culture has warped views of health as a result of our loss of the compass that was meant to keep us in balance in this crucial area.

We are swept from extreme to extreme—from pharmaceuticals to herbs, from surgery to "massaging energy flows"—because we have forgotten the fundamental instructions our Creator gave us in the Bible, which serves as a human being's operating handbook. Most people today are unaware that the true God—the Creator of the cosmos and Designer of the human body—is deeply concerned about human health because the false god of health has replaced the God of the Bible.

The Bible has several scriptures on the topic. Although some misguidedly try to turn health into a religion by becoming zealots, the fact is that biblical health ideas are significant, rational, and wonderfully useful!

The Bible is not a guide to good eating or good health. However, God gives us foundational guidelines in the Bible to help us make decisions that will advance health and ward against sickness. In ancient Israel, fundamental health education and national health policy direction were the responsibility of the priests and Levites rather than doctors, health authorities, or politicians. We'll see how straightforward and current this knowledge is when we look at some biblical health concepts, even though they were written down thousands of years ago!

The Bible contains essential facts that God revealed and that it has taken thousands of years for medical science to verify. Unfortunately, many theologians do not see the importance of the health-related lessons found in the Bible, and as a consequence, they have failed to fulfill a crucial task that God has given them.

MEATS, CLEAN AND UNCLEAN

The biblical health restrictions about clean and unclean meals are perhaps the most well-known and least understood (Leviticus 11; Deuteronomy 14). People sometimes refer to them as "Jewish" food regulations because Orthodox Jews still adhere to them, although Muslims and other people also follow corresponding dietary restrictions.

Many theologians contend that these biblical prohibitions were not intended to protect people's health, but rather to distinguish the ancient Israelites from other groups of people. Others argue that because Christians are under a New Covenant and not the Old Covenant, they are free to consume anything they like. Some claim that biblical food prohibitions are absurd and outdated and just restrict people's liberties and pleasures.

These commonly held beliefs are founded on erroneous information. The majority of theologians have little to no expertise in biology, ecology, microbiology, parasitology, epidemiology, or public health, yet understanding these subjects helps us understand the logic behind the regulations governing clean and unclean foods. Scavengers, such as snails, crabs, lobsters, and gulls, are common dirty creatures whose ecological function is to consume dead plants or animals.

Other dirty creatures, such as clams and oysters, are filter feeders whose biological function is to clean the water in lakes, streams, and estuaries. Predators like lions, snakes, and alligators are examples of other dirty creatures whose ecological function is to control the size and well-being of other animal populations. The filthy animals God created are forbidden to be used as human food for several crucial ecological reasons. They were created by God for something else.

These food limitations are also being implemented for significant health reasons. Many dirty animals are hosts to parasites that may make people sick. Pigs, bears, squirrels, and raccoons all transmit illnesses like trichinosis. Crabs and crayfish, which are scavengers, may spread lung and liver flukes. Infection rates with parasites are usually high in human communities that regularly ingest these critters.

Clams and oysters are examples of filter-feeding creatures that may be hazardous for human eating due to high levels of pathogenic bacteria, viruses, and poisonous heavy metals. You are essentially eating organisms that God designed to be nature's "clean-up crew" when you consume these critters. Would you consume the things in your trash disposal or vacuum cleaner bag? Hardly! Nevertheless, a lot of "gourmet" meals are prepared with these animals, blissfully unaware of the dangers.

The biblical rules about clean and unclean meals were inspired by a God who created all things for a purpose—a God concerned with promoting health and avoiding sickness! They were far from being antiquated Old Covenant prohibitions! A crucial first step in preventing the main parasite infections that affect hundreds of millions of people worldwide is avoiding unclean meals. We harm ourselves when we consume things that God has forbidden us to ingest. Unfortunately, contemporary theologians do not appreciate the importance of this potent public health neither do a lot of self-described Christians.

BIBLE DIETARY LAW

Other significant directives found in the Bible are ones that medical science has just lately begun to comprehend. Although Moses was inspired to write that blood and fat, even from clean animals, were forbidden to be eaten as human sustenance (Leviticus 3:17; 7:23–26; Genesis 9:4), eating "fatback," making blood sausage, and combining blood and milk are still customary practices in certain societies. Animal blood may carry germs and viruses that spread illness. This significant commandment from the Bible was created to stop the spread of disease.

Equally significant is the rule against ingesting visible fat, particularly in light of how it applies to our contemporary diet. The association between high-fat diets and heart disease, stroke, and many forms of cancer is one of the most important findings from epidemiological research undertaken in the previous 50 years.

These are the major causes of mortality in nations where fatty foods are eaten in great quantities, including burgers, French fries, triple-thick milkshakes, ice cream, and fatty salad dressings. Bacon, hot dogs, cheese, and spreads are just a few examples of familiar meals that might have fat content over 50%. Today's culture is plagued with weight issues due to high-fat and high-calorie diets. Medical research has discovered that consuming too much fat might be harmful, yet God told Moses thousands of years ago! Tragically, this scriptural knowledge has gone unrecognized for so long.

God provided humans with clean meats, fruits, vegetables, and grains for nourishment, according to the book of Genesis (Genesis 1:29; 2:16; 9:3). Whole grains, fruits, and vegetables all include fiber and other complex carbs. Only recently have nutritionists begun to understand these compounds' importance. Fiber, which was formerly disregarded, gives gut contents weight and is crucial in preventing colon cancer and other chronic disorders.

A healthy diet should also include complex carbohydrates since they help lower cholesterol levels, which lowers the risk of heart disease and stroke.

The increased intake of processed carbohydrates is yet another severe issue with Western diets. The nutrients in refined wheat and sugar have been removed. People who eat a lot of refined carbs are more likely to develop diabetes and other associated issues. But the Bible gives a warning against this kind of eating. Even Solomon was moved to write: "It is not healthy to consume much honey" (Proverbs 25:16, 27). Despite being "natural," honey is in a way "refined" by the bees that produce it. Making honey starts with pollen, which is obtained from several flowers.

The biblical advice is to consume refined carbs in moderation. But many individuals consume more than 100 pounds of refined sugar each year, again to their harm, due to the massive consumption of soft drinks (more than 50 gallons per person annually in the United States), pastries, sweets, and pre-sweetened meals.

When considered objectively, these biblical recommendations concur with the most recent dietary guidance: minimize consumption of meat and processed carbs while increasing intake of fruits, vegetables, and whole grains (see the Food Guide Pyramid published by United States governmental agencies). Since truth never changes, this is not unexpected. To benefit humans, God revealed essential nutritional truths thousands of years ago. He then handed this knowledge to religious figures so that they may pass it on to others. It is disheartening to consider that the majority of human misery might be avoided if we would just obey God's commands!

Controversial medical topics are also addressed in the Bible. Some individuals think it is improper for people to consume meat. In the ancient world, vegetarianism was encouraged by pagan Greek thinkers as well as many people in the East. Some contend that since it is not explicitly stated in Scripture that God provided meat for Adam and Eve to consume, it is inappropriate to consume it.

This, however, ignores the fact that God—the source of the rules governing clean and unclean meats—said, "These are the animals which you may eat" (Deuteronomy 14:4). Also ignored is the fact that Abraham fed two angels and the one who would later become the New Testament figure of Jesus Christ (Genesis 18:3). That supper featured milk, butter, bread, and meat (Genesis 18:3–8). Fish was presented to Jesus' followers (John 21:9–13). Paul warns New Testament believers not to be sucked into vegetarianism (Romans 14:2; 1 Timothy 4:3). The Bible was designed to assist us in maintaining our equilibrium in the face of concepts that promote excessive eating practices.

Drug and alcohol abuse

Alcohol is seen as the devil's brew by many religious people, raising a "red flag"! While the Bible expressly forbids intoxication and alcohol misuse (Proverbs 20:1; 1 Corinthians 5:11), it also encourages the use of alcohol for some other reasons (Deuteronomy 14:26). Jesus transformed wine from water at a wedding (John 2:1–11). To promote health, Paul advised drinking. Use a little wine, he advised Timothy, "for the sake of your stomach and your frequent ills" (1 Timothy 5:23). Moderation is crucial (Philippians 4:5, KJV).

The effects of moderate alcohol use include relaxation, a rise in HDL levels, a decreased risk of cardiovascular disease, and an increase in stomach acid, which helps older people with digesting. The Bible offers significant prohibitions on alcohol usage, necessitating individual choices that shape character.

Although the Bible doesn't address cigarettes or recreational drugs, it does include explicit guidelines for their usage. As stated by Paul in 1 Corinthians 6:19, "Your body is the temple of the Holy Spirit," and "If anybody defiles the temple of God [the body], God will destroy him" (1 Corinthians 3:17). The Bible makes it very clear that we are not to harm our bodies, which drug usage (regardless of whether the substance is legal or not) unmistakably does.

Anyone with common sense can realize that these biblical concepts are preventative. Indulging in alcoholic, cigarette, or drug desires is a kind of lust and idolatry, breaking many of the Ten Commandments. Biblical health guidelines are created to make sure that such joys will be beneficial and joyful experiences rather than restricting human pleasure.

ALSO, EXERCISE!

Many people have been encouraged to think throughout history that Christians need to live ideally a peaceful, sedentary life of prayer, study, and meditation. However, Jesus Christ was a carpenter at a time when there were any power tools when He arrived on our planet, not as a hermit.

He picked fishermen without diesel-powered winches to bring in their nets, including Peter, Andrew, James, and John! In Matthew 4:19, John 7:17, and Matthew 11:54, Jesus commanded His earliest followers to "follow" Him, which

included traveling hundreds of miles annually.
These instances are crucial because living an active lifestyle helped keep them healthy and gave them the energy they needed to finish their task.

Although our main attention should be on spiritual things, the apostle Paul stated that "bodily exercise benefits a little" (1 Timothy 4:8). The results of recent studies confirm this. Since its effects are primarily short-term, exercise must be done often! But these advantages—lowering cholesterol levels, blood pressure, and stress—as well as avoiding diabetes, heart disease, and a variety of other issues—are crucial.

A SPIRITUAL PERSPECTIVE

The identification of what is referred to as "spiritual health" has been one of the most fascinating breakthroughs in health education. This field of research recognizes the critical part that values and beliefs play in shaping behavior and health.

People who have a strong moral code, consistently attend church, and believe in God are less likely to smoke, misuse alcohol, or have promiscuous sexual behavior. Such behaviors are called sins in the Bible and should be avoided. The biblical prohibitions against overeating, laziness, intoxication and sexual promiscuity are just as essential for us today as the biblical dietary laws—and they align with public health recommendations for healthy living.

Compared to our permissive "if it feels good do it" society's flawed attitudes, biblical health standards present a startling contrast. People are more likely to adopt healthy practices that prevent illness when biblical principles are instilled in them by their families, churches, and schools.

However, the Bible contains more than just a guide to healthy living. While many people today have forgotten God's commands and have turned health into a goal in and of itself, the Bible offers deeper justifications for our actions.

The Bible teaches that we are fashioned in his likeness (Genesis 1:26), that we shall be judged for our deeds, and that we need to "glorify God in our bodies" (1 Corinthians 6:20). However, our bodies were not created to be eternal (Psalm 39:5;

James 4:14; Hebrews 9:27). Our greatest task is to acquire a mind like God's, a character like His, and love for others (Philippians 2:5). (John 15:17). This existence is only a practice run towards an incredible future (1 Corinthians 9:24–27).

If we learn to obey God's commands and take good care of what He has given us, we shall be rewarded with the opportunity to rule with Jesus Christ when He comes to build the Kingdom of God on earth (Revelation 5:10). The gospel is that (Mark 1:14–15)!

The believers will serve as instructors (Isaiah 30:20–21) to all of mankind, explaining the rules of God, including these crucial biblical health concepts (Isaiah 2:2–4). As a result of their work, global health will significantly improve, and "the earth will be full with the knowledge of the Lord as the rivers cover the sea" (Isaiah 11:9). (see Isaiah 35:5–7; Jeremiah 30:17). Learning to live by the biblical ideals inspired by our Creator has many compelling benefits. He is getting us ready to help Him alter the course of human history, put an end to the sickness pandemic, and advance a way of living that not only leads to bodily, mental, and spiritual health but also everlasting life!

Do not fall for a lie! Biblical religion places a high priority on health-related issues. They are vital secrets for promoting health and preventing sickness, provided by our Creator. These concepts are a tremendous benefit for all of humanity when properly understood, articulated, and put into practice. Beloved, I wish that you would thrive in all things and be in good health, just as your soul does (3 John 2).